The Ebook Title:

The Comprehensive Guide to Intermittent Fasting And How to Naturally Improve Health, Control Hunger, Shed Weight, and Slow Down Aging.

Copyright Page:

Introduction:

Intermittent fasting (IF) is presently one of the world's most prevalent health and fitness trends.

Folks are using it to lose weight, enhance their health and simplify their way of life.

Several studies show that it can have dominant effects on your body and brain and might even assist you live longer is an eating arrangement that cycles between periods of fasting and eating.

It doesn't stipulate which foods you should eat however, *when* you should eat them.

In this respect, it's not a diet in the conventional sense though more correctly defined as an eating pattern.

Common intermittent fasting ways consist of daily 16-hour fasts or fasting for 24 hours, two times per week.

Fasting has been a norm all through human evolution. Early hunter-gatherers didn't have superstores, freezers or food accessible year-round. Sometimes they couldn't get anything to eat.

Chapter1

What is intermittent Fasting?

Fasting has been practiced for thousands of years and is indispensable across many different religions and cultures around the world.

Nowadays, new ranges of fasting put a new twist on the olden practice.
16/8 intermittent fasting is one of the most prevalent styles of fasting. Protagonists state that it's a stress-free, suitable and justifiable

way to lose weight and advance overall
health.

What Is This16/8 Intermittent Fasting?

16/8 intermittent fasting comprises
restricting intake of foods and calorie-
containing beverages to a set window of
eight hours per day and refraining from food
for the remaining 16 hours.

This cycle can be repeated as often as you
like — from just once or twice per week to
every day, subject to your personal
preference.

16/8 intermittent fasting has increased
rapidly in acceptance in recent years,
particularly among those considering to lose
weight and burn fat.

Whereas other diets always set stringent
rules and regulations, 16/8 intermittent

fasting is easy to track and can offer real results with slight effort.

It's usually considered less limiting and more flexible than numerous other diet plans and can fit into just about any routine.

In addition to improving weight loss, 16/8 intermittent fasting is also understood to advance blood sugar control, enhance brain function, and promote longevity.

SUMMARY 16/8 intermittent fasting includes eating only for the duration of the eight-hour window and fasting for the remaining 16 hours. It might support weight loss, advance blood sugar, boost brain function, and enhance longevity.

Chapter 2

How to Get Started:

16/8 intermittent fasting is simple, harmless, and viable.

To get going, start by picking an eight-hour window and restrict your food intake to that period.
Many folks choose to eat between noon and 8 p.m., as this means you'll only have to fast overnight and miss breakfast though can still eat a balanced lunch and dinner, along with a few snacks all through the day.

Others elect to eat between 8 a.m. and 6 p.m., which permits plenty of time for a healthy breakfast around 8 a.m., a standard lunch around noon, and a light early dinner or snack around 5 p.m. before beginning your fast.

Moreover, you can try out and pick the time frame that best fits your schedule.
Irrespective of when you eat, it's suggested that you eat many small meals and snacks spaced equally throughout the day to help stabilize blood sugar levels and keep hunger under regulation.

Furthermore, to make the most of the most probable health benefits of your diet, it's imperative to stick to nutritious whole foods and beverages during your eating periods.

1. Filling up on nutrient-rich foods can help round out your diet and let you earn the rewards that this regimen has to offer.

Try balancing each meal with a good selection of healthy whole foods, like:
- **Fruits:** Apples, bananas, berries, oranges, pineapple, watermelon, etc.
- **Veggies:** Broccoli, cauliflower, vegetable, leafy greens, tomatoes, etc.
- **Whole grains:** Quinoa, rice, oats, barley, buckwheat, etc.
- **Healthy fats:** Olive oil, avocados coconut oil, shear butter oil

- **Sources of protein:** Meat, poultry, fish, legumes, eggs, nuts, walnuts, etc.

Drinking calorie-free beverages such as water and unsweetened tea and coffee, even while fasting, can also control your appetite while keeping you hydrated.

Nevertheless, binging or overdoing it on junk food can repudiate the positive effects connected with 16/8 intermittent fasting and might cause more harm than good to your health.

SUMMARY: To start 16/8 intermittent fasting, select an eight-hour window, and restrict your food consumption to that time. Be sure to eat a balanced, healthy diet in the course of your eating period.

How It Affects Your Cells and Hormones:

Whenever you fast, numerous things occur in your body on the cellular and molecular level.

For instance, your body regulates hormone levels to make stored body fat more available.

Your cells also initiate vital repair processes and alter the expression of genes.
Here are some alterations that happen in your body when you fast:

- **Human Growth Hormone (HGH):** The <u>levels of growth hormone</u> hit the roof, increasing as much as 5-fold. This has advantages for fat loss and muscle gain, to name just a few).

- **Insulin:** <u>Insulin sensitivity</u> enhances levels of insulin drop normally. Lower insulin levels make stored body fat more available.

- **Cellular restoration:** When fasted, your cells initiate cellular healing processes. This comprises autophagy, where cells digest and eliminate old and dysfunctional proteins that build up inside cells.

Gene expression: There are variations in the function of genes associated with long life and shield against disease

A Very Dominant Weight Loss Tool:

Weight loss is the most usual reason for folks to try intermittent fasting ().
By making you eat fewer meals, intermittent fasting can lead to an instant reduction in calorie ingestion.
Moreover, intermittent fasting changes hormone levels to enable weight loss.
In addition to reducing insulin and raising growth hormone levels, it increases the discharge of the fat-burning hormone norepinephrine (noradrenaline).

Because of these variations in hormones, short-term fasting may raise your metabolic rate by 3.9–16% ().

Intermittent fasting causes weight loss by altering both sides of the calorie equation by making you eat fewer and burn more calories.

Studies show that intermittent fasting can be a very potent weight-loss tool.

A 2019 review study found that this eating pattern can cause 4–9% weight loss over 3–26 weeks, which is a substantial amount, equated to most weight loss studies .

According to a similar study, individuals also lost 5–8% of their waist circumference, showing a considerable loss of damaging <u>belly fat</u> that builds up around your organs and causes disease.

Another study revealed that intermittent fasting causes less muscle loss than the more usual method of continuous calorie restriction.

Conversely, keep in mind that the foremost reason for its achievement is that intermittent fasting assists you eat fewer calories generally. If you binge and consume vast amounts during your eating periods, you might not lose any weight at all.

SUMMARY
Intermittent fasting may marginally enhance metabolism while assisting you to eat fewer calories. It's a very efficient way to lose weight and belly fat.

Chapter3

Benefits of 16/8 Intermittent Fasting:

16/8 intermittent fasting is a popular diet since it's stress-free to follow, flexible, and viable in the long term.

It's also expedient, as it can cut down on the amount of time and money you require to spend on cooking and making food each week.

In terms of health, 16/8 intermittent fasting has been connected with a long list of benefits, comprising:

- **Enhanced weight loss:** Limiting your intake to a few hours per day helps cut calories over the day, though studies also show that fasting could enhance metabolism and increase weight loss.

, intermittent fasting can assist you to lose weight and belly fat, short of having to limit calories deliberately

- (**Better blood sugar control**: Intermittent fasting has been found to lessen fasting insulin levels by up to 32% and lower blood sugar by 4–7%, possibly reducing your risk of diabetes.

- **Improved longevity**: However, evidence in humans is restricted. Some animal studies have established that intermittent fasting might extend longevity.

  SUMMARY16/8 intermittent fasting is cool to follow, flexible, and desirable. Animal and human studies recommend that it might increase weight loss, advance blood sugar levels, augment brain function, and extend longevity.

- **Inflammation:** Some researches show decreases in indicators of inflammation, a key driver of several chronic diseases (

- **Heart health:** Intermittent fasting could reduce "bad" LDL cholesterol, blood triglycerides, inflammatory markers, blood sugar, and insulin resistance, all of which are risk features for heart disease.

- **Cancer:** Animal studies advocate that intermittent fasting may avert cancer.

- **Brain health:** Intermittent fasting intensifies the brain hormone BDNF and may help the growth of new nerve cells. It may also guard against Alzheimer's disease

- **Anti-aging:** Intermittent fasting can prolong lifespan in rats. Studies revealed that fasted rats lived 36–85% longer).

- Keep in mind that the research is still in its infant stages. Many of the studies were small, short-term, or piloted in animals. Several questions have yet to be answered in higher quality human studies.

•

Drawbacks of 16/8 Intermittent Fasting

16/8 intermittent fasting may be connected with numerous health benefits, but it does have some downsides and may not be right for everyone.
Hunger is the foremost side effect of intermittent fasting.

You may also feel weak, and your brain may not function as well as you're used to.
This may only be momentary, as it can take some time for your body to familiarize yourself with the new meal schedule.

If you have a medical condition, you should ask your doctor before trying intermittent fasting.
This is mainly significant if you:
- Have diabetes.
- Have difficulties with blood sugar control.
- Have low blood pressure.
- Take medicines.
- Are malnourished.

- Have a history of eating disorders.
- Are you a woman who is trying to get pregnant?
- Are you a woman with a history of amenorrhea?

Are you expectant or breastfeeding? Limiting your consumption to just eight hours per day can cause some persons to consume more than usual during eating periods in an attempt to compensate for hours spent fasting.

This might lead to weight gain, digestive difficulties, and the development of unwholesome eating habits.

16/8 intermittent fasting might also cause short-term adverse side effects when you're first getting in full swings, such as hunger, weakness, and fatigue — yet, these typically subside once you get into a routine.

Moreover, some study advocates that intermittent fasting could affect men and women differently, with animal studies reporting that it could hinder fertility and reproduction in females.

Conversely, more human studies are needed to assess the effects that intermittent fasting might have on reproductive health.

In any case, be sure to start slowly and ponder stopping or consulting your doctor if you have any worries or experience adverse symptoms.

SUMMARY Controlling daily food intake might lead to weakness, hunger, improved food intake, and weight gain. Animal studies show that intermittent fasting might influence men and women in a different way and may even affect fertility.

Chapter 4

Is 16/8 Intermittent Fasting Right for You?

16/8 intermittent fasting could be a sustainable, safe, and secure way to advance your health when paired with a nutritious diet and a healthy lifestyle.
Conversely, it shouldn't be seen as a substitute for a balanced, well-rounded diet rich in whole foods. Not to mention, you can still be in good physical shape even if intermittent fasting doesn't work for you.

Although 16/8 intermittent fasting is usually considered safe for most healthy adults, you should talk to your physician before giving it a try, particularly if you have any underlying health conditions.
This is important if you're taking any medicines or have diabetes, low blood pressure, or a history of disordered eating.

Intermittent fasting is also not recommended for women who are trying to conceive or those who are expectant or breastfeeding.
If you have any worries or experience any adverse side effects when fasting, be sure to consult your physician.

The Bottom Line:

16/8 intermittent fasting comprises eating only during an 8-hour window and fasting for the remaining 16 hours.
It might support weight loss and improve blood sugar, brain function, and longevity.
Eat a healthy diet during your eating period and drink calorie-free beverages such as water or unsweetened teas and coffee.
It's better to have heart-to-heart with your doctor before trying intermittent fasting, particularly if you have any underlying health conditions.

Should Women Fast?

There is some proof that intermittent fasting may not be as useful for women as men.
For instance, one study indicated that it enhanced insulin sensitivity in men, but then worsened blood sugar control in women.

However, human studies on this topic are unavailable, studies in rats had found that intermittent fasting could make female rats skinny, masculinized, infertile and cause them to miss cycles.

 (There are many unreliable reports of women whose menstrual period stopped when they began doing IF and went back to usual when they restart their other eating pattern.

For these reasons, women should be cautious with intermittent fasting.
They should follow distinct guidelines, like easing into the practice and stopping instantly if they have any difficulties like amenorrhea (absence of menstruation).
Consider holding off on intermittent fasting if you have issues with fertility and are trying to get pregnant.

This consumption pattern is usually also a lousy notion if you're pregnant or breastfeeding.

Chapter 5

Seven ways to do intermittent fasting

Therc are several different means of intermittent fasting. The techniques vary in the number of fast days and calorie allowances.

Intermittent fasting comprises wholly or partially refraining from eating for a set amount of time before eating frequently again.

Some studies propose that this way of eating may offer benefits like fat loss, better health, and increased longevity. Protagonists assert that an intermittent fasting program is stress-free to uphold than traditional, calorie-controlled diets.

Each person's experience of intermittent fasting is separate, and diverse styles will suit different individuals.

In this part of the ebook, we will discuss the most popular kinds of intermittent fasting and provide guidelines on how to maintain this sort of diet.

There are several methods of intermittent fasting, and folks will choose different styles. Read on to discover about seven different ways to do intermittent fasting.

1. **Fast for 12 hours a day**:

Different styles of intermittent fasting may suit different persons.
The guidelines for this diet are simple. Any person needs to choose and stick to a 12-hour fasting window every day.
According to some scientists, fasting for 10–16 hours could make the body burn its fat

stores into energy, releasing ketones into the bloodstream. This should add to weight loss.

This sort of intermittent fasting plan might be an excellent opportunity for beginners. This is because the fasting window is relatively small, much of the fasting takes place during sleep, and the person can ingest the same number of calories each day.

The best way to do the 12-hour fast is to take account of the period of sleep in the fasting window.

For illustration, an individual could elect to fast between 8 p.m. and 8 a.m. They would require to finish their dinner before 8 p.m. and wait up until 8 a.m. to eat breakfast; however, they would be asleep for much of the time in between.

Fasting for 16 hours

Fasting for 16 hours a day, leaving an eating gap of 8 hours, is termed the 16:8 method or the Lean gains diet.
All through the 16:8 diet, men usually fast for 16 hours each day, and women fast for

minimum of 14 hours. This sort of intermittent fast may be useful for someone who has previously used the 12-hour fast though, did not see any benefits.

On this fast, people usually finish their evening meal by 9 p.m. and then miss breakfast the next day, not eating again up until noon.

Research on mice states that limiting the feeding gap to 9 hours protected them from obesity, inflammation, diabetes, and liver disease, even when they consumed the same total number of calories as mice that ate whenever they desired.

Fasting for 2 days a week:

Persons following the 5:2 diet eat reasonable amounts of healthful food for 5 days and lessen calorie consumption on the other 2 days.
In the course of the 2 fasting days, men usually consume 650 calories and women 550 calories.

Typically, individuals separate their fasting days in the week. For instance, they might fast on a Monday and Thursday and normally eat on the other days. There should be at least 1 non-fasting day inserted between fasting days.

There is restricted research on the 5:2 diet, which is also acknowledged as the Fast diet. A study concerning 108 overweight or obese women found that limiting calories two times weekly and continuous calorie restriction led to comparable weight loss. The study also found that this diet lessens insulin levels and enhanced insulin sensitivity among partakers.
A small-scale study observed the effects of this fasting style in 27 overweight women. For one menstrual cycle, the women lost 6.0. percent of their body weight and 9.0 percent of their overall body fat.

Conversely, these measurements returned to normal for most of the women after 7 days of regular eating.

Alternate day fasting:

There are numerous variations of the alternate-day fasting plan, which comprises fasting every other day.

For some individuals, alternate day fasting means a comprehensive evading of solid foods on fasting days, whereas other folks permit up to 550 calories. On feeding days, people always select to eat as much as they want.

One research state that alternate-day fasting is effective for weight loss and heart health in both healthy and overweight adults. The scientists found that the 34 participants lost an average of 5.3 kilograms (kg) or over 12 pounds (lb), over 14 weeks.

To a certain extent, alternate day fasting is an extreme form of intermittent fasting, and it might not be appropriate for novices or those with certain medical conditions. It might also be problematic to sustain this type of fasting in the long term.

A weekly 24-hour fast:

On a 24-hour diet, a person can have teas and calorie-free drinks.

Fasting entirely for 1 or 2 days a week, recognized as the Eat-Stop-Eat diet, consist

of eating no food for 24 hours at a time. Several persons fast from breakfast to breakfast or lunch to lunch.
Folks on this diet plan could have water, tea, and other calorie-free drinks in the course of the fasting period.
People should return to regular eating patterns on the non-fasting days. Eating lessens a person's total calorie consumption; however, but does not limit the particular foods that the individual consumes.

A 24-hour fast can be baffling, and it might lead to fatigue, headaches, or irritability. Several individuals find that these effects become less extreme over time as the body changes to this new eating pattern.

Folks might profit from trying a 12-hour or 16-hour fast before moving to the 24-hour fast.

Meal skipping

This flexible tactic to intermittent fasting may be excellent for beginners. It includes intermittently missing meals.
People can choose which meals to avoid according to their level of hunger or time

restraints. Conversely, it is essential to eat healthful foods at each meal.

Meal skipping is expected to be most fruitful when individuals monitor and respond to their body's hunger signals. Folks using this style of intermittent fasting will eat when they are hungry and miss meals when they are not.
This may look more natural for some persons than the other fasting methods.

The Warrior Diets

The Warrior Diet is a moderately extreme form of intermittent fasting.
The Warrior Diet consists of eating very little, typically just a few servings of raw fruit and vegetables, in the course of a 20-hour fasting window, then eating one large meal at night. The eating window usually is only around 4 hours.
This form of fasting may be suitable for people who have tried other methods of intermittent fasting already.

Followers of the Warrior Diet claim that humans are natural nocturnal eaters and that eating at night permits the body to gain nutrients in line with its circadian rhythms. All through, the 4-hour eating phase, people should make sure that they ingest plenty of vegetables, proteins, and healthful fats. They should also consist of some carbohydrates.

Even though it is conceivable to eat some foods during the fasting period, it can be thought-provoking to stick to the strict guidelines on when and what to eat in the long term. Also, some people struggle with eating such a large meal so close to sleep time.

There is also a danger that people on this diet will not eat sufficient nutrients, such as fiber. This could increase the risk of cancer and have an adverse effect on digestive and immune health.

Instructions for sustaining intermittent fasting:

Yoga and light exercise may well help to make intermittent fasting stress-free.
It can be thought-provoking to stick to an intermittent fasting program.

The following instructions could help people stay on track and take full advantage of the benefits of intermittent fasting:

- Staying hydrated. Drink plenty of water and calorie-free drinks, like herbal teas, all through the day.
- Shunning obsessing over food. Strategize sufficiently of distractions on fasting days to avert thinking about food, like catching up on paperwork or going to a movie house.
- Resting and relaxing. Shun vigorous activities on fasting days, though light exercise like yoga, may be helpful.

- Making every calorie count. If the selected plan permits some calories for the duration of the fasting period, select nutrient-dense foods rich in protein, fiber, and healthful fats. Instances consist of beans, lentils, eggs, fish, nuts, and avocado.

- Consuming high-volume foods. Choose to fill yet low-calorie foods, which contain popcorn, raw vegetables, and fruits with high water content, namely grapes and melon.

- Increasing the taste short of the calories. Season meals generously with garlic, herbs, spices, or vinegar. These foods are particularly low in calories, yet they are packed of flavor, which may help reduce feelings of hunger.

- Selecting nutrient-dense foods after the fasting period. Eating high fiber, vitamins, minerals, and other nutrients helps keep blood sugar levels steady and avoid nutrient deficiencies. A balanced diet will also add to weight loss and general health.

There are many different ways of intermittent fasting, and there is no single plan that will work for everyone. Individuals will experience the best results if they try out the various styles to see what suits their lifestyle and preferences.

Regardless of the type of intermittent
fasting, fasting for extended periods when
the body is unprepared can be problematic.

These forms of dieting may not be suitable
for everyone. If a person is prone to
disordered eating, these approaches may
exacerbate their unhealthy relationship with
food.
People with health conditions, including
diabetes, should speak to a doctor before
attempting any form of fasting.

For the best results, it is essential to eat a
healthy and balanced diet on non-fasting
days. If necessary, a person can seek
professional help to personalize an
intermittent fasting plan and avoid pitfalls.

Chapter 6

Frequently Asked Questions on Intermittent Fasting:

These are solutions to the most common questions about intermittent fasting

Q:

Are all forms of intermittent fasting styles safe?

A:
People have practiced fasting for thousands of years, however its safety rest on more on who is doing the fasting than the style of fasting itself.
People who have malabsorption, are in danger of low blood sugar, or have other medical conditions should look for the guidance of their healthcare provider.

Whereas most persons can securely practice many fasting styles, extreme sorts of intermittent fasting, such as the Warrior Diet, could lead to insufficient intake.

Can I Drink Liquids In the course of the Fast?

Absolutely. <u>Water</u>, <u>coffee</u>, <u>tea</u>, and other non-caloric beverages are okay. Do not add sugar to your coffee. Small amounts of milk or cream may be okay.
Coffee can be most useful during a fast, as it can blunt hunger.

Isn't It Unwholesome to Miss Breakfast?

No. The problem is that most conventional <u>breakfast skippers</u> have an unhealthy way of life. If you make sure to consume healthy food for the rest of the day, then the practice is perfectly healthy.

Can I Take Supplements While Fasting?

Yes. Conversely, keep in mind that some supplements such as fat-soluble vitamins may work better when taken with meals.

Can I Work out While Fasted?

Yes, fasted workouts are excellent. Some people recommend taking branched-chain amino acids (BCAAs) before a fasted workout.
You can find many BCAA products on Ecommerce stores

5. Will Fasting Cause Muscle Loss?

All weight loss methods can cause muscle loss, so it's essential to lift weights and keep your <u>protein intake</u> high. One study showed that intermittent fasting causes less muscle loss than regular calorie restriction ().

6. Will Fasting Slow Down My Metabolism?

No. Studies show that short-term fasts boost metabolism (). However, longer fasts of 2 or more days can <u>subdue</u> metabolism).

7. Should Kids Fast?

Permitting your child to fast is perhaps a bad idea.

Of nutrients such as fiber, vitamins, and minerals. Thus, people should approach this style of fasting with restraint.
Intermittent fasting – a two-word combination that was used only sporadically *(see what I did there?)* 12 years ago, and now it looks like everybody is talking about it.

Even my 84-year-old grandma has told me she is "on" it.
Google search popularity for the word "intermittent fasting" in the last 12years
However, if you are reading this ebook, you are one of the thousands of folks each day who want to learn and comprehend what the big fuss is about finally.

Maybe, even try it yourself? Well, you came to the right place. We've been helping people lose thousands of pounds and kilos via our Fasting challenges and meal plans.

And before I begin with all the info, I just love to say thank you for reading this ebook. I sincerely hope after reading this; you will be **completely ready to start the Intermittent Fasting journey yourself.**

Intermittent fasting is an act of fasting intermittently. It is an eating arrangement where you cycle between periods of eating and periods of voluntary fasting over the course of the single day, week, or another well-defined period.
Huh?

In human terms, it merely means monitoring when do you eat and when you don't. When you don't eat any food or drinks (besides water), you are termed a fasting window. And the rest is titled…eating window.

How long you select to have your fasting or eating window is genuinely up to you and your preferred Intermittent Fasting plan. I will talk about all the most current schedules and their pros and cons.

HOW DOES INTERMITTENT FASTING WORK?

The power of Intermittent Fasting (IF) comes in two forms and shapes: caloric limitation (eating fewer calories than you require) and lessen meal frequency (how many meals/snacks you eat per day).

An *average adult* would have breakfast at 7 am, lunch at noon, snack at 4 pm, dinner at 8 pm and then an "I can't go to bed being hungry"-sort-of-snack at 11.30 pm.

That's five meals over the course of 15.30s hours, and if you don't track a stringent portion control – you'll most likely eat more calories than you spent that day, which will lead to gaining extra weight.
Moreover, your body will be working all that time digesting the food and will not have sufficient time for so-needed recovery activities.

When following any intermittent fasting plan, you are reducing the meal frequency all through your day, making it merely harder to consume 3 big meals and 2 snacks within twice or even less time (and please don't try to prove me wrong).

All of these outcomes in a lower chance of going overboard with your calorie consumption and also more time for the body to achieve recovery operations such as autophagy.

SCIENCE OF INTERMITTENT FASTING FOR WEIGHT LOSS

To comprehend the science of intermittent fasting, we need to look into the fundamentals of nutrition.
And it is very straight-forward: the food we consume gets broken down to molecules and ends up in our blood, which feeds the cells in our bodies.
Part of those molecules are net carbohydrates (all carbs in the meal minus the fiber), and our body converts them into sugar (glucose), so our cells may well use it for energy.

To be able to use sugar for the energy we require insulin, which gets formed in our pancreas each time we throw in some food with carbohydrates.
Any leftover sugars that we don't ingest get stored in the form of fat with the knowledge that we will use that fat for energy later, as soon as, we have no sugar left.

The best way how NOT to end up having enormous fat reserves (and becoming overweight) is to expend the same amount of energy you get from food.
Furthermore, life is not perfect, and many of us have lifestyles that reduce our chances of moving all through the day. Conversely,

office workers used to spend 80% of their waking hours sitting.

Thus, what can we do to lose or not gain weight?

One way to do it is to concentrate on increasing your energy intake through increased physical activity or in layman's terms – working out and doing sports. Though, you knew this one already, didn't you?

Another way though is to concentrate on consuming less food than you require for the energy that day and, as a result, forming a caloric deficit.

And that's where intermittent fasting comes in.

Intermittent fasting makes it easier to lessen the number of meals and calories you consume per day. It's a lot more expedient to not eat at all for some time vs. eating less *(I refuse to trust people who say they could eat just one cookie)*.

Chapter 7

IS INTERMITTENT FASTING SAFE AND HEALTHY?

Certainly, intermittent fasting does have a lot of advantages. We talk about them in this ebook.
In general, Intermittent Fasting is safe for most persons, though, you have to know the hazards.

It is also an excellent time to say that this ebook should and does not aim to replace advice from your physician. You should often refer to your physician before planning any fasting and notably extended fasting (longer than 24h).

Nowadays, that we made it clear, these are some of the cases (though might not be restricted to) that does not go well with intermittent fasting:

§ if you have a diabetes
§ if you take drugs for blood pressure or
heart disease
§ if you are heavy with child or
breastfeeding
§ if you have a history of disordered eating
§ if you don't sleep well
§ if you are below 18 years old

Also, you should be a lot more careful if you
are keen to prolonged fasting, which reliant
on the source you follow will be continuous
fasting for either anything more than 24, 48,
or 72 hours. There is a general agreement
that any fasts more extended than 72 hours
should be done under the strict guidance of
medical supervision.

HOW TO START & HOW TO DO INTERMITTENT FASTING

One of the reasons I usually think
Intermittent Fasting took over is how stress-
free it is to start it.

Factually, the only thing you should adopt before you begin is which Intermittent Fasting schedule type you are planning to follow.

And before you make this choice, it is imperative to comprehend the various types of Intermittent Fasting. That's how you will find the one that works the best for you and fits your unique way of life.
For your convenience, these are the **most common Intermittent Fasting Schedules.**

KINDS OF INTERMITTENT FASTING

INTERMITTENT FASTING 16/8

How: Fast for 16 h and Eat 8 h
By following this **16/8 Intermittent Fasting Schedule**, you fast for 16 hours and limit your eating to an 8-hour eating window.
It is actually up to you which you will select 16 out of 24 hours to limit yourself from eating. You can elect to have an eating

window from 8 am to 4 pm, 10 am to 6 pm, noon to 8 pm, or any other plan, as long as it is 16h of unbroken non-eating.

The majority of the persons who follow this plan, choose to miss breakfast rather than dinner, though different people have different life rhythms.

What's great, that out of 16h, you'll perhaps be sleeping at least 7-9 of them; thus, we're just talking about 9-8h of fasting each day.

It's also worth saying that we have faith in the Intermittent Fasting 16/8 method is the most viable and stress-free to start with, Lastly, if you're looking for the **meal plans to go along the 16/8 Intermittent Fasting plan**, you can get them here.

INTERMITTENT FASTING 18/6

How: Fast for 18 h and Eat 6 h

Almost the same to the one above, if you select **the 18/6 Intermittent Fasting**

Schedule, you should fast for 18 hours and limit your eating to a 6-hour eating window. It's merely two more hours of fasting every day, though, for a beginner faster, these 2 hours can make all the changes.

That's why we suggest starting with 16/8 for at least a month then moving to 18/6 because you'll have a much more pleasant start, and that's a critical element between quitting and not.
Slow and steady wins the race – take it easy and pay attention to your body before going extreme.

INTERMITTENT FASTING 5:2 A.K.A THE FAST DIET

How: 2 days per week limit calories to 550-650, 5 days per week eat ordinarily
5:2 Intermittent Fasting lets you usually eat 5 days per week and limits your calorie intake to 550-650 per day during the other 2 days.

When selecting your fasting days, keep in mind that there should be at least one regular eating day in between.

Please note, that your results depend on what you eat during the 5 days of non-fasting, therefore, stick to the nutritious and whole diet all through for max results.

INTERMITTENT FASTING 20/4 A.K.A. WARRIOR DIET

How: Fast for 20 h and Consume for 4h

In contrast to other methods, while following the **20/4 Intermittent Fasting Schedule,** you are permitted to eat some raw fruits and vegetables and some lean protein during the 20 hr fast period.

This fasting period is based on the knowledge that our ancestors spent their days hunting and gathering and would feast at night. Hence, the 4-hour eating window will be in the evening, and you should follow a distinct order of eating precise food groups: beginning with vegetables, proteins and fat, and eating carbs only if you are still hungry.

OMAD FASTING - ONE MEAL A DAY A.K.A 23 /1

How: Fast for 23h and eat one time a day
Another typical fasting plan is termed one-meal-a-day (OMAD).
It is precisely what it sounds like – you select a time in a day that is the most appropriate for you to have your on and only meal of the day.

I know what you're thinking – isn't that almost starving? And yes, you are very right – OMAD diet shouldn't be done without thought on how to get at least 1250 calories during that one meal.

Therefore, if you elect this 23/1 fasting – make sure your meal is a hearty and nutritious one.
If you're keen to try out OMAD – there is a **7-day challenge** that is packed with all the info you need and also comprises meal ideas and recipes to make it super easy...

24 HR FAST A.K.A. EAT STOP EAT

How: Fast for 24 h 1-2 times a week

While following 24 hours fast (make accessible by Eat Stop Eat method, you should fast for 24 hours 1-2 days a week and normally eat on other days. That way, you should lessen overall calorie ingestion by ca 10% and henceforth lose weight.

CIRCADIAN RHYTHM FASTING:

How: Begin fasting when the sun goes down and start eating when the sun goes up You might have heard that our bodies have been planned to follow Circadian rhythm – an internal clock that runs 24h each day and controls our energy levels based on the rhythm of the day and night.

Therefore, if you follow Circadian Rhythm fasting, you would let daylight to decide your hours.

As soon as the sun is up – your eating window begins. As soon as it is down and it gets dark – you should commence your Fasting.
The only downside of it is that the success of it depends on where you live. In some places on our Planet Earth such as northern Norway, the sun never sets for 76 days in a year, and that's a fasting period that we certainly don't suggest.

EXTENDED A.K.A. PROLONGED FASTING

How: Fast for more than 24 hours once a month

As stated before, extended or lengthy Fasting typically means anything between 24 and 96 hours of Fasting.
It is not suggested to do it more frequently than once a month, and anything above 48-

72h of Fasting should be done under a doctor's observation.

Indeed, there are lots of individuals who don't follow this suggestion and nothing happens; however, it is dangerous, and, we **do not** suggest it if you are not experienced faster and particularly if you have any of the medical conditions described above.

.

SUGGESTED INTERMITTENT FASTING PLAN FOR NOVICES

We often propose starting with the most common and beginner-friendly method – **Intermittent Fasting 16/8.**
, we suggest easing into Intermittent Fasting by beginning with 12h of Fasting and 12h of eating and adding one fasting hour each day till you reach the anticipated 16/8 schedule.

Note: 16/8 also occurs to be the most prevalent method among celebrities. If you are interested in knowing how they practice fasting and what are the main benefits (*Coldplay* vocalist Chris Martin even believes Intermittent Fasting assist him in singing better!),.

WHAT TO CONSUME DURING INTERMITTENT FASTING

A widespread misconception is that you can permit yourself to eat anything while doing Intermittent Fasting, comprising fast food, sugary and highly treated dishes. If you aim to lose weight, advance productivity and get healthier, it is vital to stick to healthy meals.

This means eating whole foods and shunning the typical suspects like sugar, processed foods, empty carbs, etc.
The kind of diet you select is up to you; as long it is well-balanced and fits your way of life. For many, the Keto Diet has been recognized to be a great supplement to Intermittent Fasting, as it may aid you to burn more fat.

WHAT TO DRINK DURING INTERMITTENT FASTING

To get all the health benefits of Intermittent Fasting like fat loss, improved metabolic rate, lower blood sugar levels, boost in the immune system and others, you have to limit from consuming any caloric food.

Though, you can still drink non-caloric beverages since they do not break your fast and permit you to get all the benefits of Fasting.

This is because non-caloric beverages do not cause the release of insulin, and as a result, do not impede with fat burning and autophagy (cellular cleanup).

This would compose:

§ Water
§ Sparkling water
§ Mineral water
§ Plain black coffee
§ Plain tea

NEED ASSISTANCE TO TRACK YOUR INTERMITTENT FASTING?

Sometimes technology can be our best friend and help us stick to our commitments. If you require extra support or merely want to make your life stress-free, there are many intermittent fasting apps accessible on the market to help you out.

We have studied several apps and made our list of **the best 6 Intermittent Fasting apps:**

§ Do Fasting
§ Life Fasting Tracker
§ Fasten
§ Simple Fasting Tracker
§ Fasting Tracker
§ Zero

TIPS

It is necessary to uphold a reliable eating time. Being steady with your plan has proven to produce better results,

Chapter 8
INTERMITTENT FASTING PLAN: 7-DAY DAILY GUIDE

To assist you kick-off your Intermittent Fasting journey in a stress-free, fun and workable way, we arranged a 21 Day Intermittent Fasting Plan that offers you action for each day, with a full description and more learnings.

Scroll down and see a preview of the first 7 Intermittent Fasting days. If you feel like it's time to take matters in your own hands and make Intermittent Fasting a workable lifestyle,

DAY 1

TODAY'S TASK: 12 h Fast | 12 h Eat
TODAY'S MISSION: Select your Intermittent Fasting schedule
All through the first week, you want to ease into your intermittent Fasting gradually. This is why we propose starting with 12 hours of fasting on your first day, and steady go up to 16 hours on Day 5, by adding 1 extra hour of fasting each day.

That way, it is easier for your body and brain to get used to the new method of eating; also, you give yourself more time to get used to Intermittent Fasting.

On your first day, we also want you to select the **Intermittent Fasting schedule** that fits your lifestyle best, and that you will stick to it in the course of the entire 7-day Intermittent Fasting Challenge. Consistency has proven to be one of the most contributing factors to success,

DAY 2

TODAY'S TASK: 13 h Fast | 11 h Eat
TODAY'S TASK: Study the fundamentals of Intermittent Fasting
On Day 2, you will be extending your fast to 13 hours. Just one extra hour likened to yesterday – you could do it!

Day 2 is splendid to get you introduced into the healthy eating guiding principle that will sustain your Intermittent Fasting objectives: just focus on eating more whole foods and shunning the typical suspects like sugar, processed foods, empty carbs etc.

We will offer you a list of usual meals and foods you could eat to get better Intermittent Fasting results. Think simple though lovely and balanced meals you could do at home, like poached eggs with spinach, meatballs with zucchini noodles, feta cheese salad or home-grown hummus for a snack.

DAY 3

TODAY'S TASK: 14 h Fast | 10 h Eat
TODAY'S MISSION: Describe your rewards
Rewards are vital when launching your new Intermittent Fasting routine. Henceforth on Day 3, we want you to **state your rewards for each successfully fasted day**.

Why are rewards so significant?

A reward drives a positive signal to your brain, saying "Doing this feels good, we

should do more of it!". It could be anything that makes you feel good.
Preferably, the **finest Intermittent Fasting reward** should be associated with your fundamental needs for relaxing, mingling, food or playing.

Or, your incentive could also be a simple (but influential!) celebratory action you do instantly after concluding the habit like encouraging yourself up and saying "Good job" or indicating yet another day off of your daily progress tracking sheet you get when joining the 7-day challenge.

If the reward is higher, for instance, dinner at a pricey, however, so pleasant restaurant, you can try token method – e.g., each successful day fasting "gives you" 2 tokens. Whenever you have collected 6 symbols, you get to treat yourself and go out to the cafeteria.

DAY 4

TODAY'S TASK: 15 h Fast | 9 h Eat
TODAY'S ASSIGNMENT: Prepare a high protein lunch

On Day 4 of Intermittent Fasting, you will be fasting for 15 hours before now! To break your fast, we propose having a high protein lunch, which will back your weight loss objectives.

For instance, you could make yourself steamed or grilled veggies with a protein of your choice, like grilled meat, poultry, fish, tofu, eggs, beans, legumes or nuts, and seeds.

DAY 5

TODAY'S TASK: 16 h Fast | 8 h Eat
TODAY'S WORK: Drink black coffee when hungry
On Day 5 of Intermittent Fasting Plan, you will finally be getting your decisive **16/8 Intermittent Fasting plan** of fasting for 16 hours and eating inside 8 hours window. And… it will genuinely be pretty easy to attain, something we have seen ourselves and in hundreds of folks that already took the7 Day Intermittent Fasting challenge.

To aid you to go through the 16 hours of Fasting and limit your hunger, in case you are witnessing one, we suggest drinking black coffee. It is packed full of antioxidants and is appetite suppressing, too (do not overdo it though!).

Keep in mind: **Intermittent Fasting coffee is black coffee.** The implication, don't add any sugar, milk or creamers to it – no cappuccino, latte or flat white, only black coffee.

If you need to have something sweet, add natural sweetener stevia, then be careful as it might bring about hunger.
Not a coffee drinker? Go for black or green tea or a glass of water.

DAY 6

TODAY'S TASK: 16 h Fast | 8 h Eat
TODAY'S MISSION: Go for a walk
Are you eager to lose some pounds during these 7 fasting days? It is imperative to stick to a healthy diet, and we also suggest integrating some exercise in your routine.

Go for a **walk just before you break your fast**. Even a quick 25 min walk will do the magic.
Walking is a great way to advance your overall fitness, your mood and simply get some fresh air. Most fundamentally, going for a walk will switch your attention from hunger and assist you in passing those last hours of fasting easier.

DAY 7

TODAY'S TASK: 16 h Fast | 8 h Eat
TODAY'S MISSION: Go for a walk
These days, keep your new 16/8 Intermittent Fasting Schedule, and while doing so, reflect on your progress from the week.

Reflecting on your progress is part of success – to do so, take a full-body photo, record your weight and liken them with your starting weight and photo. You should start seeing the first outcomes in your weight and physical appearance.
Moreover, we want you to answer a couple of questions to reflect on your progress, such as how do you feel, if you have witnessed changes in your energy,

mood and skin from Intermittent Fasting, etc.

Going through an exercise like that will assist you to recognize where, and most significantly, why you could be struggling and therefore will aid you to take actions to fast-track your results and make intermittent fasting a new workable habit.

.

16:8 intermittent Fasting, which individuals sometimes call the 16:8 diet or 16:8 plan, is a common type of Fasting. Folks who follow this eating plan will fast for 16 hours a day and eat all of their calories during the remaining 8 hours.

Anticipated benefits of the 16:8 plan consist of weight loss and fat loss, as well as the prevention of type 2 diabetes and other obesity-associated conditions.

.

Chapter 8

What is 16:8 Intermittent Fasting?

Most persons on a 16:8 intermittent fasting plan elect to ingest their daily calories during the middle part of the day.

16:8 intermittent Fasting is a type of time-restricted Fasting. It includes consuming foods during an 8-hour window and shunning food, or fasting, for the remaining 16 hours each day.
Some people are of the view that this method works by supporting the body's circadian rhythm, which is its internal clock.

Most folks who follow the 16:8 plan refrain from food at night and for part of the morning and evening. They tend to ingest their daily calories during the middle of the day.

There are no limitations on the kinds or amounts of food that a person can eat in the

course of the 8-hour window. This
flexibility makes the plan comparatively
easy to follow.
How to do it
The easiest way to monitor the 16:8 diet is
to select a 16-hour fasting window that
comprises the time that a person devotes to
sleeping.

Some professionals advise finishing food
ingestion in the early evening, as
metabolism slows down after this time.
Conversely, this is not possible for
everyone.
Some individuals may not be able to eat
their evening meal until 8 p.m. or later. Even
so, it is best to shun food for 2–4 hours
before bed.

People may select one of the following 8-
hour eating windows:
- 9 a.m. to 5 p.m.
- 8 a.m. to 4p.m.
- midday to 8 p.m.
-

In this timeframe, people can consume their
meals and snacks at appropriate times.
Eating frequently is essential to avert blood

sugar peaks and dips and to shun excessive hunger.

Some folks might need to try out to find the best eating window and mealtimes for their way of life.

Suggested foods and tips:

While the 16:8 intermittent fasting plan does not stipulate which foods to eat and shun, it is helpful to emphasis on healthful consumption and to limit or ignore junk foods. The eating of too much unhealthful food might cause weight gain and contribute to disease.

A balanced diet concentrates mainly on:

- fruits and vegetables, which could be fresh, frozen, or preserved (in water)
- whole grains, comprising quinoa, brown rice, oats, and barley
- lean protein sources, like poultry, fish, beans, lentils, nuts, seeds, low-fat cottage cheese, and eggs

- health-giving fats from fatty fish, olives, olive oil, coconuts, avocados, nuts, and seeds

-

Fruits, vegetables, and whole grains are very high in fibre, so they can assist in keeping a person feeling full and fulfilled. Healthful fats and proteins can also contribute to satiety.

Beverages can play a part in satiety for those participating in the 16:8 intermittent fasting diet. Drinking water often all through the day can help lessen calorie intake because people frequently mistake thirst for hunger.

The 16:8 diet plan allows the ingesting of calorie-free drinks — such as water and unsweetened tea and coffee — during the 16-hour fasting window. It is essential to consume fluids habitually to avoid dehydration.

Tips

People may find it easier to stick to the 16:8 diet when they follow these guidelines:

- Drinking cinnamon herbal tea all through the fasting period, as it may subdue the appetite
- consuming water frequently all through the day
- Watching less television to lessen exposure to images of food, which may fuel a sense of hunger
- Exercising just before or during the eating window, as exercise can trigger hunger
- practicing mindful eating when consuming meals
- Trying contemplation during the fasting period to permit hunger pangs to pass

Health benefits:

Researchers have been studying intermittent Fasting for decades.
Study outcomes are sometimes conflicting and inconclusive. Moreover, the research on intermittent Fasting, comprising 16:8 Fasting, shows that it may offer the following benefits:

Weight loss and fat loss:

Eating during a set period can aid people to decrease the number of calories that they ingest. It may also help enhance metabolism. A 2019 study proposes that intermittent Fasting leads to more significant weight loss and fat loss in men with obesity than ordinary calorie restriction.

Research from 2019 reports that men who followed 16:8 tactics for 9 weeks while resistance training showed a reduction in fat mass. The partakers sustained their muscle mass all through.

In contrast, a 2020 study found very little change in weight loss between participants who practised Intermittent Fasting — in the form of alternate-day Fasting rather than 16:8 Fasting — and those who lessen their overall calorie intake. The dropout rate was also high among those in the intermittent fasting assembly.

Chapter9

Disease prevention

Supporters of intermittent Fasting recommend that it can avert several conditions and diseases, comprising:

- type 2 diabetes
- heart conditions
- some cancers
- neurodegenerative diseases
-

Conversely, the research in this area remains restricted.

A 2019 review reports that intermittent Fasting shows promise as a substitute for traditional calorie restriction for type 2 diabetes risk reduction and weight loss in folks who have overweight or obesity.

The scientists caution, though, more research is needed before they can reach reliable conclusions.
A 2019 study shows that in addition to weight loss, an 8-hour eating window might

help lessen blood pressure in adults with obesity.

Other studies state that intermittent Fasting decreases fasting glucose by 4–7% in those with prediabetes, even though it does not affect healthy persons. It may also lessen fasting insulin by 12–58% after 3 to 26 weeks of Intermittent Fasting. Time-restricted Fasting, like the 16:8 method, may also safeguard learning and memory and slow down diseases that disturb the brain.

A 2019 annual review notes that animal research has specified that this form of Fasting decreases the risk of nonalcoholic fatty liver disease and cancer.

Lengthy life span:

Animal studies recommend that intermittent fasting may help animals live longer. For instance, one study found that short-term, repeated Fasting enhanced the life span of female mice.

The National Institute on Aging points out that, even after years of research, scientists still cannot clarify why Fasting may prolong life span. As a result, they cannot authorize the long-term safety of this practice.

Human studies in the area are limited, and the possible benefits of intermittent Fasting for long human life are not yet known.

Side effects and risks:

16:8 intermittent Fasting has some related risks and side effects. As a consequence, the plan is not right for every person.
Potential side effects and risks consist of:
- hunger, weakness, and tiredness in the opening stages of the plan
- overeating or eating unhealthful foods in the course of the 8-hour eating window due to extreme hunger
- heartburn or reflux as a consequence of overeating

Intermittent Fasting may be less helpful for women than men. Some study on animals advocates that intermittent Fasting could adversely affect female fertility.
Persons with a history of disordered eating may wish to shun intermittent Fasting. The National Eating Disorders Association caution that Fasting is a risk factor for eating disorders.

The 16:8 plan may also not be appropriate for those with a history of depression and anxiety. Some research specifies that short-term calorie restriction might get rid of depression; however, that chronic calorie restriction can have the opposite effect.
More research is required to comprehend the implications of these findings.
16:8 intermittent Fasting is inappropriate for those who are pregnant,
breastfeeding, or trying to get pregnant.

The National Institute on Aging concluded that there is insufficient proof to suggest any fasting diet, particularly for older adults.

Individuals who want to try the 16:8 method or other kinds of intermittent Fasting should talk to their doctor first, specifically if they are taking medications or have:

- an underlying health condition, like diabetes or low blood pressure
- a history of disordered eating
- a history of mental health disorders

Anyone who has any worries or experiences any adverse effects of the diet should see a physician.

Diabetes

While evidence shows that the 16:8 method may be useful for diabetes prevention, it may not be right for those who already have the condition.

The 16:8 intermittent fasting diet is not suitable for folks with type 1 diabetes. Conversely, some people with prediabetes or type 2 diabetes may be able to try the diet under a medic's supervision.

People with diabetes who wish to go for the 16:8 intermittent fasting plan should see their doctor before making modifications to their eating habits.

Summary

16:8 intermittent Fasting is a common form of intermittent Fasting. Potential benefits comprise weight loss, fat loss, and a decrease in the risk of some diseases. This diet plan may also be easier to follow than other forms of Fasting. People doing 16:8 intermittent Fasting should concentrate on eating high fibre whole foods, and they should stay hydrated all through the day.

The plan is not right for everyone. Individuals who wish to go for the 16:8 intermittent fasting diet should speak to a dietitian if they have any concerns or underlying health conditions.

What is Intermittent Fasting?

"Conventional wisdom" isn't that smart. We're going to take two extensively accepted healthy eating "rules" and turn them on their head:

RULE #1: You HAVE to eat first thing in the morning:
Make sure you begin with a healthy breakfast so that you could get that metabolism firing first thing in the morning!
"Eat breakfast just like a king, lunch such as a prince, and dinner like a pauper."

There are even studies that show those that eating earlier in the day lose more weight than those who ate later in the day or missed a meal.

RULE #2: Consume lots of small meals for weight loss. Make sure you eat at least six small meals during the day, so your metabolism stays operating at maximum capacity all day long."

In other words, "consume breakfast and lots of small meals to lose weight and get perfect health."

Conversely, what if there are science and research that shows MISSING BREAKFAST (the horror! blasphemy!) can help with optimal human performance, mental and physical health improvement, maximum muscle retention, and body fat loss?

That's where an Intermittent Fasting Plan comes in.

Intermittent Fasting is not a diet, but somewhat a *dieting pattern*.

In simpler terms: it's making a mindful decision to miss individual meals on purpose.

By fasting and then eating on purpose, intermittent Fasting usually means that you ingest your calories in the course of a specific window of the day, and select not to consume food for a longer window of time.

There are a few different techniques to take advantage of Intermittent Fasting, which I got from Lewis over at <u>Lean Gains</u>, a resource precisely built around fasted strength training:

INTERMITTENT FASTING 16/8 PLAN
What it is: Fasting for 16 hours and then only eating within a particular 8-hour window. For instance, only eating from noon-8 PM, basically missing breakfast. Some persons only consume in a 6-hour window or even a 4-hour window. This is "feasting" and "fasting" parts of your days and the most common method of Intermittent Fasting. It's also my favored method (5 years running).

Two illustrations: The top means you are missing breakfast, the bottom means you are skipping dinner each day:

You can alter this window to make it work for your life:

· **If you start eating at** 8 AM, stop eating and start fasting at 4 pm.

· **If you start consuming at** 11 AM, stop eating and start fasting at 8 pm.

· **If you start eating at** 3 PM, stop eating and start fasting at 11 pm.

· **If you begin eating at** 6 PM, stop eating and start fasting at 2 AM.

INTERMITTENT FASTING 24 HOUR PLAN:

Miss two meals one day, where you take 24 hours off from eating. For instance, eat on a usual schedule (concluding dinner at 8 PM) and then you don't eat again until 8 PM the following day.

With this plan, you eat your usual 3 meals per day, and then sometimes choose a day to skip breakfast and lunch the next day.

If you can merely do an 18 hour fast, or a 21 hour fast, or a 22 hour fast – that's satisfactory! Adjust with different time frames and see how your body reacts.

Two illustrations: missing breakfast and lunch one day of the week, and then another where you miss lunch and dinner one day, two days in a week.

Note: You could do this once a week, two times a week, or whatsoever works best for your life and condition.

In other words, both those weekly charts above come from our Intermittent Fasting Plan.

Most folks struggle with knowing precisely when to eat and when to halt eating, and sticking with it.

Bottom of Form
Those are the two most common intermittent fasting plans, and the two we'll be concentrating on, although there are many variations of both that you can alter for yourself:
· Some persons eat in a 4-hour window; others do 6 or 8.
· Some folks do 20-hour fasts or 24-hour fasts.

· Another approach is to eat only <u>one meal a day (OMAD)</u>.
You'll need to experiment, alter it to work for your lifestyle and goals, and see how your body reacts.

How Does Intermittent Fasting Work?

Now, you might be feeling: "okay, thus by skipping a meal, I will eat less than I usually eat on average (2 meals in place of 3), and therefore I will lose weight, right?"
Yes.
By cutting out a whole meal each day, you are eating fewer calories per week – even if your two meals per day are somewhat more significant than before. Mostly, you're still ingesting fewer calories per day.

In this sample, you're consuming LARGER lunches and dinners than you usually do, but then, by skipping breakfast, you'll ingest 550 fewer calories per day.
And hence, weight loss!

This is underscored in a contemporary JAMA study in which both calorie limited

dieters and intermittent fasters lost related amounts of weight over a year.
That doesn't tell the FULL story, as the timing of meals can also impact how your body responds.

Intermittent Fasting can assist since your body operates in a different way when "feasting" likened to when "fasting": Whenever you eat a meal, your body uses a few hours processing that food, burning what it can from what you just expended. Since, it has all of this readily-available, easy to burn energy (thanks to the food you consumed), your body will select to use that as energy rather than the fat you have stockpiled.

In the course of the "fasted state" (the hours in which your body is not consuming or break down any food) your body doesn't have a freshly consumed meal to use as energy.

Therefore, it is *more likely* to pull from the fat stockpiled in your body as it's the only energy source enthusiastically accessible. *Burning fat = win.*

The same goes for working out in a "fasted" state.
Short of a ready supply of glucose and glycogen to pull from (which has been dwindling throughout your fasted state, and hasn't yet been restocked with a pre-workout meal), your body is forced to adjust and pull from a source of energy that it does have accessible: the fat stored in your cells.

Why does this work?

Our bodies respond to energy ingestion (eating food) with insulin production.
The more sensitive your body is to insulin, the more possible you'll be to use the food you consume resourcefully, and your body is most susceptible to insulin following a period of Fasting.

These changes to insulin production and sensitivity can help lead to weight loss and muscle creation

Next: Your glycogen (a starch stockpiled in your muscles and liver that your body can burn as fuel when needed) is exhausted during sleep (aka for the duration of Fasting), and will be depleted even further in the course of training, which can lead to improved insulin sensitivity.

This means that a meal following your workout will be used more effectively: transformed to glycogen and stored up in your muscles or burned as energy instantly to help with the recovery process, with insignificant amounts stored as fat.

Liken this to a typical day (no intermittent fasting): With insulin sensitivity at normal levels, the carbs and foods consumed will see packed glycogen stores and sufficient glucose in the bloodstream, and hence be more probable to get stored as fat.

Back to Fasting: Growth hormone is amplified in the course of fasted states (both during sleep and after a period of Fasting). Combine this enhanced growth hormone secretion: the reduction in insulin production (and hence increase in insulin sensitivity), and you're preparing your body for muscle

growth and fat loss with intermittent
Fasting.

The less science-y version: Intermittent
Fasting can assist in teaching your body to
use the food it ingests more efficiently,

and your body can study to burn fat as fuel
when you rob it of new calories to regularly
pull from (if you consume all day long).

TL/DR: For several different physiological
reasons, Fasting can help boost weight loss
and muscle building when done
appropriately.

I know Intermittent Fasting can be crushing
for many, which is why we write this ebook
with to help people to understand what's
going on, and how to make it work for
THEIR life.
If that sounds like you,

Should I Eat 6 Small Meals a Day?

There are a few main reasons why diet books suggest six small meals:

> **1) When you consume a meal, your body *does* have to burn additional calories merely to process that meal.** Thus, the theory is that if you eat all day long with small meals, your body is always burning extra calories, and your metabolism is firing at maximum capacity, right? Well, that's not true.

Whether you eat 2050 calories, spread out all through the day, or 2200 calories in a small window, your body will burn the equivalent number of calories processing the food.

Thus, the whole "keep your metabolism firing at optimum capability by often eating" sounds good in principle; however, reality tells a different story.

When you eat smaller meals, you *might* be less probable to overeat in the course of your regular meals. I can certainly see some truth here, particularly for people who struggle with portion control or don't know how much food they should be eating.

Conversely, once you teach yourself and take control of your eating, some might find that eating six times a day is very prohibitive and needs a lot of effort. I know I do. Likewise, because you're ingesting six small meals, I'd say that you perhaps never feel "full," and you might be MORE probable to eat extra calories in the course of each snack.

Though grounded in apparently logical philosophies, the "six meals a day" doesn't work for the reason you think it would (#1), and typically only works for people who have problem with portion control (#2). If we think back to caveman days, we'd have been in serious trouble as a species if we *had* to eat every four hours. Do you think Joe Caveman pulled out his pocket sundial six times a day to feed his likewise portioned meals?

Hell no! He consumed when he could, endured and dealt with extended periods of NOT eating (no refrigeration or food storage). His body adapted to function optimally still sufficient to go out yet and catch new food.

A new study (written about in the NYT, underscored by <u>LeanGains</u>) has done an excellent job of challenging the "six-meals-a-day" method for weight loss:

There were [no statistical] alterations between the low- and high- [meal frequency] groups for adiposity indices, appetite extents or gut peptides (peptide Y.Y. and ghrelin) either previously or after the intervention. We say that increasing meal frequency does not stimulate more significant body weight loss under the conditions defined in the present study.

Factor in the impending physiological benefits itemized in the preceding section, and you got yourself some known proper science-backed proof to ponder trying Intermittent Fasting if you want to reduce body fat and build muscle.

Chapter 10

Should I Try intermittent Fasting? (6 Things to Consider)

Nowadays, that we're finished a lot of the science stuff, let's get into the reality of the condition: why should you contemplate Intermittent Fasting?

#1) Since it can work for your goals. Though we know that not all calories are fashioned equal, caloric restriction plays a dominant role in weight loss.

When you fast, you are also making it stress-free to limit your total caloric intake over the week, which can lead to steady weight loss and maintenance.

#2) Because it simplifies your day. Rather than having to make, pack, eat, and the time your meals every 2-4 hours, you just skip a meal or two and only care about eating food in your eating window. It's one less choice you have to make every day.

It could permit you to relish bigger portioned meals (hence making your taste buds and stomach satiated) and STILL eat fewer calories on average.

#3) It needs less time (and possibly less money). Rather than having to prepare or buy three to six meals a day, you only have to make two meals.
In place of stopping what you're doing six times a day to consume, you just only have to stop to eat twice. Rather than having to do the dishes six times, you only have to do them two times.
Rather than having to buy six meals a day, you only have to purchase two.

#4) It encourages more energetic insulin sensitivity and improved growth hormone secretion, two secrets for weight loss and muscle gain. Intermittent Fasting helps you make a double whammy for weight loss and building a solid figure.

#5) It can level up your brain, comprising counteracting conditions such as Parkinson's, Alzheimer's, and dementia.
As elucidated here in this TEDx talk by Mark Mattson, a professor at Johns Hopkins University and Chief of the Laboratory of Neurosciences at the National Institute on Aging, Fasting is grounded in serious research, and more studies are coming out showing the benefits:

#6) Plus, Wolverine does it: